HOW TO LOWER YOUR CHOLESTEROL LEVEL FAST AND NATURALLY

Fast and natural low density lipoprotein regulation

Julius Abdul

Disclaimer

It is not a complete guaranty that the recommendation in this book will lower your cholesterol, nor is it intended to replace your medical treatment.

You are aware that a consultation with a qualified healthcare professional, such as your doctor, is not intended to be substituted by reading this book. To be sure you are in good health and that following the information in this book won't hurt you, you should speak with your doctor or another qualified healthcare professional before starting any health modification program or altering your lifestyle in any manner, if after reading the information, you develop any strange symptoms.

THE A TO Z OF CHOLESTEROL SUMMARIZED; EVERYTHING YOU NEED TO KNOW ABOUT HDL AND LDL

The Hidden Secretes About Cholesterol

TABLE OF CONTENT

Introduction

When People Hear The Word Cholesterol, They Are Always Filled With Anxiety And Fear That It Will Clog Their Arteries. As A Result, They Get Tested For Cholesterol And Become Alarmed When Their Result Is High. However, The Following Are The Facts Regarding Cholesterol:

The Majority Of The Cholesterol In Your Body Is Produced Internally; Daily, Your Body Produces 3,000 Milligrams Of Cholesterol. This Cholesterol Is Not Derived From Your Food, As Nearly Every Cell In Your Body Produces Cholesterol. It Is Split As Follows: Your Body Cells Make Up The 2,000, while your liver produces the remaining 1,000. You will probably agree that this level of cholesterol is excessive given that it is the same as a pound of butter, fourteen eggs, or three hundred strips of bacon.

Given that eating more causes your body to produce less cholesterol and eating less causes your body to produce more, the real issue here should be, "Why does your body make this much cholesterol if it's so bad?" To set the record straight, cholesterol is not what is represented by HDL (high-density lipoprotein) or LDL (low-density lipoprotein). Keep in mind that All LDL and HDL are High or Low Density "Lipoprotein" (the word "protein" is stressed).

While LDL is the cholesterol that travels from your liver to the body and is thought to be harmful but is not, HDL is a protein shuttle that transports cholesterol from the body, specifically the cholesterol leaving the arteries and returning to the liver.

In summary, while cholesterol is often feared for its potential to clog arteries, it's crucial to understand that the body internally produces the majority of it. The daily production, equivalent to a pound of butter, prompts the question of why the body generates such quantities if cholesterol is deemed harmful. Importantly, cholesterol is not solely represented by LDL or HDL; both are lipoproteins with distinct roles. LDL transports cholesterol from the liver to the body, while HDL acts as a shuttle, moving cholesterol from arteries back to the liver. This nuanced perspective challenges the simplistic good versus bad narrative surrounding cholesterol.

Why Is Cholesterol Necessary?

Well, your body has a trillion cells, and of those cells, around half of their membranes are composed of cholesterol. These membranes include the structure of your brain and neurological system, as well as the myelin sheath that surrounds the nervous system.

Now, let's talk about cell membranes; It is involved in the production of bile, which is a detergent that aids in breaking down fat to assimilate essential fatty acids and fat-soluble vitamins. This is why you need cholesterol to make vitamin D and bile to help you absorb vitamins A, E, and K2, which are all necessary for soluble vitamins that you need, but you cannot make bile to extract them from the food that you eat without cholesterol. It is permeable and allows nutrition electrolyte molecules to travel out of the cell, protecting the cells against microbes and foreign viruses.

Because the body needs the hormones to respond to stress, cholesterol is produced in greater amounts when under stress. This is because cholesterol is a raw material precursor for adrenal hormones. Sex hormones: progesterone, estrogen, and testosterone are produced from cholesterol. This is why statin medications cause side effects in men, such as decreased libido, and in women, complications with progesterone, estrogen, and testosterone.

A low-cholesterol diet can cause dysfunctional myelin, which is the lipid layer surrounding the nervous system in the brain, and exacerbate the condition. In addition, cholesterol feeds the immune system, which requires it to function, in part because the immune system's control over white blood cells depends on the adrenal gland's production of cortisol.

Because one of the functions of LDL is to neutralize toxins from bacteria in the cell, cholesterol is necessary to fight infection and counteract the toxic effects of bacteria. LDL cholesterol is regarded as the bad cholesterol. Although it is present at the crime scene, it is the good cholesterol trying to cure an ulcer or lesion. This leads people to believe that LDL is bad when, in fact, it is the good guy. After all, why would your body consider producing it if it is harmful?

In essence, the purpose of cholesterol is to produce more cortisol during stressful situations like surgery or the winter months when the body produces more of these hormones to adjust to the changing weather. Therefore, if your cholesterol is elevated, always question why rather than taking medication to lower it.

In summary, Cholesterol is crucial for cell membranes, brain structure, and myelin sheath. It's vital for bile production, aiding fat and vitamin absorption. Cholesterol is a precursor for hormones, including those responding to stress and sex hormones. A low-cholesterol diet can harm the nervous system. Cholesterol supports the immune system and is necessary for fighting infection. LDL, considered "bad," is essential for neutralizing toxins. Elevated cholesterol may be a natural stress response; questioning it is crucial before medication.

Atherosclerosis Plaque

The majority of the time, people believe that the artery-clogging plaque is a large piece of cholesterol, as cholesterol is bad and causes heart attacks and strokes. However, let's look at what this plaque is. Did you know that collagen-containing fibrous plaque makes up roughly 68% of plaque? Keep in mind that we are not against collagen and have never encountered anyone who believes it to be harmful. Only 16% of the plaque is made up of lipids, and of those 16%, 74% are unsaturated fat. Calcium makes up 8% of it, white blood cells, which produce the inflammatory response, make up 1%, and foam cells, or immune cells, move like trash. It indicates that cholesterol is not the cause of your clogged artery, disproving the theory that it is. As cholesterol is a healer, it responds to an attack-like ulcer by trying to apply a band-aid. Rather than questioning why, we jump to the conclusion that cholesterol is exclusively harmful to us, not realizing that it can also be beneficial.

In summary, plaque in arteries is mainly collagen (68%), not cholesterol. Only 16% is lipids, mostly unsaturated fat. Cholesterol responds to artery damage like a band-aid, challenging the belief that it's solely harmful.

Cholesterol deficiency

You know how it's always been believed that you should drastically reduce your cholesterol because it will block your arteries and is so dangerous? Well, the truth is that low cholesterol causes far more issues than high cholesterol. Do you know that if your total cholesterol is high, your chance of having a heart attack is only 0.1%? That is one-tenth of one percent. Would you take the medication if I told you that you have a one-tenth of one percent chance of having a heart attack due to your high cholesterol? Most likely not.

Low cholesterol can lead to several health issues such as depression, cancer, strokes, and aortic dissection, which is a condition in which the aorta divides and causes internal bleeding. Suicidal tendencies (this occurs because hormone production requires cholesterol), Eligible for infection, elevated risk of HIV/AIDS, raise the likelihood of developing an allergy or asthma (taking vitamin D can help with both allergies and asthma, as it functions similarly to unique cholesterol).

As a result, there are many more issues with low cholesterol than there are with high cholesterol. In 1994, low cholesterol was defined as 160 or below. However, in the present, people are attempting to lower their cholesterol to 110 and believe that this is beneficial.

In summary, low cholesterol poses more risks than high cholesterol. A total cholesterol of 110 is now considered beneficial, but low levels can lead to depression, cancer, strokes, aortic dissection, suicidal tendencies, infection susceptibility, and increased risk of allergies and asthma. High cholesterol's heart attack risk is only 0.1%.

Foods that are highest in cholesterol

If you want to elevate your cholesterol, these meals will help your body produce more cholesterol for normal functioning:

Brain

With 20% of its mass being made up of cholesterol, the brain is thought to contain some of the highest levels of cholesterol in the body. Because cholesterol is necessary for the synthesis of cell membranes and the insulation of nerve fibers, it is crucial for the brain's correct operation.

Organ Meat

Dietary cholesterol is abundant in organ meats like liver and kidney. Compared to muscle meat like chicken or beef, these meats have higher cholesterol content. It is possible for eating organ meats to raise your cholesterol. Organ meats, such as the liver and kidney, are excellent sources of cholesterol and are also high in cholesterol.

Caviar

Caviar the roe of sturgeon fish, is known for its high cholesterol content. It is a delicacy and can be a significant source of dietary cholesterol if consumed regularly.

Cod Liver Oil

Cod liver oil is extracted from the livers of codfish and is a concentrated source of cholesterol. It is also rich in omega-3 fatty acids, which can have various health benefits.

Egg yolk

Egg yolks are well-known for their cholesterol content. While egg whites are a source of protein, the yolk contains a significant amount of cholesterol. However, recent research has suggested that dietary cholesterol from eggs may not have as large an impact on blood cholesterol levels as previously thought.

Butter

Butter is a dairy product that contains cholesterol. It was a commonly consumed source of dietary fat in the past, but it has been somewhat replaced by other fats and spreads in modern diets.

Cold water fish

Certain cold water fish like salmon, mackerel, and herring, contain cholesterol, but they are also rich in heart-healthy omega-3 fatty acids, which can help lower bad cholesterol levels.

Lard

Lard is a type of animal that contains a significant amount of cholesterol. It was once a common cooking far but has largely been replaced by vegetable oils in modern cooking.

It is important to note that while these foods are high in cholesterol, the relationship between dietary cholesterol and blood cholesterol is complex. Some people are more sensitive to dietary cholesterol than others. Additionally, the idea that high dietary cholesterol directly leads to high blood cholesterol and heart disease has evolved, and it's now recognized that other factors, such as saturated and trans fats in the diet. Play significant roles in heart health.

As mentioned, a cholesterol deficiency can lead to problems as well, as cholesterol is vital for various bodily functions. Balancing your diet and consulting with a healthcare professional is crucial to maintaining optimal cholesterol levels and overall health.

In summary cholesterol-rich foods include brain, organ meats (liver, kidney), caviar, cod liver oil, egg yolk, butter, cold-water fish (salmon, mackerel, herring), and lard. While high in cholesterol, the link between dietary and blood cholesterol is complex. Some people are more sensitive, and other factors like saturated fats play a role. Maintaining a balanced diet and consulting with a healthcare professional are essential for optimal cholesterol levels.

Is Low-Density Lipoprotein (LDL) Bad?

You must understand that LDL is not the same as cholesterol, and that water does not mix with fat when it moves through the body. As a result, the body produces LDL and HDL, which are tiny particles, shuttles, or vehicles that carry cholesterol.

While high-density lipoprotein (HDL) travels from the circulatory system back to the liver to be recycled or eliminated, low-density lipoprotein (LDL) is seen as harmful since it is the cholesterol that travels from the liver to the vascular systems and then to the cells. You must comprehend this because it explains how the two proteins cooperate to exchange blood lipids, such as cholesterol and triglycerides, back and forth.

As you may already be aware, the body produces roughly 3000 mg of cholesterol daily—that's the same as the cholesterol found in 14 eggs, 300 bacon strips, or roughly one pound of butter. The body uses this cholesterol as a raw material to create cell membranes, which make up half of all the cells in the body and the total number of cells in the body is approximately 100 trillion. For this reason, the body requires a significant amount of cholesterol since it is a component of the membrane surrounding each cell, which facilitates the exchange of nutrients, vitamins, minerals, glucose, and other essential substances back and forth.

Additionally, cholesterol serves as an antioxidant, preventing damage from free radicals and having anti-inflammatory properties. It is also the precursor or building block for vitamin D. Bile is produced by the body to aid in the breakdown of fat and the extraction of fat-soluble vitamins from food, both of which are dependent on cholesterol and are necessary for life. Additionally, cholesterol is needed to produce the stress hormone cortisol as well as sex hormones such as testosterone, estrogen, and progesterone.

These are the typical roles of cholesterol, but it also performs other, lesser-known roles. For example, cholesterol reacts to emergencies by binding and inactivating bacterial toxins, which causes an increase in cholesterol levels in those who are infected. It serves as a band-aid and shields against microbial harm. this is due to the presence of the endothelium layer in the cell membrane, which surrounds the inside of blood vessels and has tiny pores that allow white blood cells and nutrients to be exchanged back and forth. Thus, cholesterol acts as a band-aid to repair injuries like lesions and ulcers.

In summary, LDL is not cholesterol itself but a carrier that transports cholesterol. It moves from the liver to cells, seen as potentially harmful. The body produces about 3000 mg of cholesterol daily, crucial for cell membranes, nutrient exchange, antioxidant function, vitamin D, bile production, and hormone synthesis. Cholesterol also acts as a band-aid in emergencies, binding toxins and repairing injuries. Understanding LDL's role is vital in comprehending how it cooperates with HDL in lipid exchange.

The types of LDL

The terms "type-A and B" refer to the two (2) forms of Low-Density Lipoprotein (LDL), and conventional cholesterol testing frequently fails to distinguish between the two. The "type A" is large buoyant, meaning that its size and fluff allow it to float. It's a normal low-density lipoprotein (LDL) because it doesn't clot or crack the epithelial wall.

However, because "type B" LDLs are dense and tiny, they can pass through the epithelial wall and begin to play a role in the creation of plaque. As a result, people who have heart attacks or strokes are more likely to have "Type B" LDLs (complications such as greater oxidation and build-up plaque). In your body, "Type A" typically lasts two days, and "Type B" lasts roughly five days, meaning it lasts longer. How can you now distinguish between these different kinds of LDL?

If you'd want, you can take the more advanced test, but examining the triglycerides and HDL is the quickest and most straightforward method of determining or distinguishing between these forms of low-density lipoproteins. If your HDL is low and your triglyceride % is high, you probably have more "Type B" LDL; conversely, if your HDL is high and your triglyceride percentage is low, you likely have more "Type A" LDL. This is the most straightforward method of determining the sort of low-density lipoprotein that you have.

In summary, two types of LDL exist - "Type A" is large and doesn't clot, while "Type B" is dense and can contribute to plaque. Standard cholesterol tests often don't differentiate. To distinguish, examine HDL and triglycerides; low HDL and high triglycerides suggest "Type B," while high HDL and low triglycerides suggest "Type A."

What types of food will increase the type A or B LDL?

Those high in saturated fats are known to raise "Type A" low-density lipoproteins (LDLs), while those high in refined sugar, carbs, and regular sugar raise "Type B" LDLs. Because people generally eat cars, this explains why almost all patients' blood evaluations performed in the lab always have high triglycerides and low HDL. However, if you consume more saturated fat, you may have high LDL, but a "Type A" that wouldn't pose any issues.

It is important to note that "Type B" LDL is not meant to be an attack; rather, it is meant to heal the lesion, inflammation, and bacteria causing it. Because it is a part of the chain reaction, it can have negative effects because the body doesn't consider long-term solutions, instead regulating its internal arsenal to solve the issue immediately however, in an attempt to heal the injury, the body creates a lot of "Type B" LDL, which then grows larger and larger. This is similar to how scar tissue forms to heal a sprained ankle or broken joint, even though its function is to stop motion and protect the area. This explains why a build-up of "Type B" LDL causes heart attacks and strokes. To decrease this, you must alter your diet to exclude foods that promote "Type B" LDL and allow your body to absorb nutrients that promote "Type A" LDL.

In summary, saturated fats increase "Type A" LDL, while refined sugar, carbs, and regular sugar raise "Type B" LDL. "Type B" LDL is produced to heal but can lead to issues if there's a buildup. To reduce it, avoid foods promoting "Type B" LDL and favor those supporting "Type A" LDL.

Why would someone have high LDL (pattern B)?

Several factors can contribute to the presence of high LDL (Pattern B) in the body:

Sugar: Remember what we said earlier sugar creates inflammation which is very destructive to the cells that is why diabetics have a lot of nerve damage, vision problems, inflammation coronary and heart disease, so sugar and refined cabs are bad.

Low thyroid: Low thyroid function can lead to elevated levels of cortisol, a stress hormone. Elevated cortisol levels can increase the production of Pattern B LDL, contributing to cardiovascular risk.

Consumption of Vegetable Oils and Trans Fats: Vegetable oils high in omega-6 fatty acids, such as soybean oil and corn oil, can promote inflammation in the body. Additionally, trans fats, which are often found in partially hydrogenated fats, can raise Pattern B LDL levels and increase the risk of heart disease.

Low Vitamin C Levels: Vitamin C plays a role in protecting blood vessels and preventing oxidative damage. Low levels of vitamin C can result in weakened blood vessels, making them more susceptible to damage and the formation of Pattern B LDL.

Glycation: Glycation is the result of combining glucose, fructose, and protein with fat or protein. For example, if you take barbecue sauce, cut it into pieces, and bake it at a temperature of about 248 degrees Fahrenheit, you will get glycation. This means that the combination of sugar and protein enters the body in a sticky form and begins to raise pattern B levels in addition to causing other problems.
It works the same way when sugar is added to deep-fried foods like doughnuts or French fries. Glycation is usually produced when you bake or cook food that has been combined with sugar fat and protein.

Consuming high fructose corn syrup, refined fructose, or large amounts of fructose can accelerate glycation by ten times since these sugars mix inside your body and can also be internal.

Surgery: Because LDL is a healer and tries to enter the body like an ambulance to help cure things, surgery will increase pattern B. However, individuals use statins to limit without realizing why LDL is necessary.

Visceral Fat: Visceral fat is linked to an increased risk of Pattern B LDL and builds up around the abdominal organs. This particular LDL subtype can arise as a result of inflammation and metabolic abnormalities that are exacerbated by visceral obesity.

The reason for all these about cholesterol is to understand LDL, what it is and what it is not and use it as an indicator to find out why it might be high and if it is higher, it could be normal if the triglycerides are normal and HDL is normal, but if the indicators are not so then you might want to know why it is higher, why you have hypothyroid issues, am I eating too much sugar or did I just got them from surgery trauma?

In summary, high LDL (Pattern B) can be caused by factors such as sugar, low thyroid function, vegetable oils/trans fats, low vitamin C, glycation, surgery, and visceral fat. Understanding these factors helps interpret LDL levels and address potential underlying issues like inflammation, metabolic abnormalities, or surgical trauma.

Conclusion

The prevailing fear surrounding cholesterol oversimplifies its role in the body. Cholesterol is predominantly produced internally, contributing to vital functions like cell membrane structure, hormone synthesis, and immune system support. While cholesterol is often associated with heart health, a nuanced understanding reveals its multifaceted benefits. LDL and HDL, both lipoproteins, play distinct roles in lipid exchange. Differentiating between "Type A" and "Type B" LDLs is crucial, with dietary choices influencing their levels. Atherosclerosis plaque is primarily composed of collagen, challenging the misconception that cholesterol is the main culprit. Furthermore, low cholesterol poses more risks than high cholesterol, and a balanced diet is essential for optimal health. Finally, understanding the factors contributing to high LDL (Pattern B) allows for a more informed approach to interpreting cholesterol levels and addressing potential underlying issues.

7 FOODS THAT LOWER BAD CHOLESTEROL (LDL) FAST AND NATURALLY

Fast and natural low density lipoprotein regulation

Introduction

Ever get the impression that the cholesterol narrative is far more complicated than what we've been told? According to conventional thinking for many years, having high blood cholesterol levels is exceedingly harmful and can cause heart attacks, strokes, and even death. It must therefore be decreased by whatever means required. These methods include reducing your intake of cholesterol and saturated fat as well as using prescription medications that lower your cholesterol. Sounds familiar?

Well, some people stopped and asked a few straightforward questions: Isn't the human body much more complicated than this oversimplified answer suggests? Doesn't our health depend on multiple markers, such as total cholesterol? How and why did cholesterol come to be the bad guy? These are the important questions that I will address for you in this book.

It is true that cholesterol is generated as a result of some key factors and part of the factors that contribute to increase in cholesterol level in the blood vessel is your gene, this is what determine how your body processes the fat you eat and your family history. Familial hypercholesterolemia is a genetic condition that results in extremely high blood cholesterol levels and early heart disease. There is a 50% probability that you will also have familial hypercholesterolemia if one of your parents does.

Another aspect that needs careful attention is excess body weight, which raises the risk of high cholesterol.

Consuming alcohol excessively might raise cholesterol levels. Alcohol has calories in it that will cause you to gain weight.

The amount of cholesterol in the body is significantly influenced by age. The likelihood of having elevated cholesterol is higher in older adults. Women typically have lower cholesterol levels than men their age before menopause. This is so that women can metabolize the extra fat needed for pregnancy and delivery. However, the hormones stop secreting after menopause, which alters how a woman's body handles cholesterol.

Regular physical activity and exercise help your body burn fat and lower cholesterol levels. Sedentary behavior increases the likelihood of having elevated cholesterol.

Choosing the wrong foods can raise your cholesterol. The appropriate ones, though, might support bringing it back down to a healthy level. All the cholesterol your body requires is produced by your liver. However, some foods, particularly those heavy in saturated fat, might raise your blood cholesterol levels. The walls of your blood vessels can develop a waxy material from excess cholesterol. This hinders or lowers blood flow, which causes a wide range of issues.

Other illnesses like diabetes, liver disease, renal disease, polycystic ovarian syndrome, and circumstances that increase female hormones like pregnancy can also result in high cholesterol levels.

These are the principal contributors to cholesterol. You'll see that many of them are lifestyle variables if you pay great attention. You need to adopt more healthy behaviors and alter your lifestyle if you want to control your cholesterol. Let's discuss the seven foods that will reduce your LDL (bad) cholesterol.

What is cholesterol?

It is like a molecule that resembles wax and is produced in the liver, cholesterol can be found in the blood and all of the body's cells. Although it is not entirely bad, your body uses it to create hormones, vitamins, and new cells. Cholesterol can be divided into two fundamental categories, these are the High-Density Lipoprotein (HDL) and the Low-Density Lipoprotein (LDL).

High-Density Lipoprotein (HDL), also known as good cholesterol, takes in and transports cholesterol back to the liver, which ultimately excretes it from the body. HDL cholesterol reduces the risk of heart disease and stroke, but LDL, or bad cholesterol, has a high-calorie content that leads to obesity, diabetes, and heart disease.

There are also two different LDL varieties, but let's talk about cholesterol first. Since cholesterol cannot float down the bloodstream and is all fat soluble, it cannot mix with water. Therefore, when your blood profile reports your total cholesterol, you must understand that what they are measuring is all the cholesterol in the various protein shuttles, primarily HDL and LVL. There are other shuttles as well, but just keep in mind that these are the two main ones.

When you see a medical report of total cholesterol, what you're seeing is a combination of the cholesterol in the

LDL and the HDL in general. Therefore, when we discuss HDL, which is known as the good cholesterol, we are referring to the HDL cholesterol that is moving from the arteries or cells back to the liver, and the LDL, which is regarded as the bad cholesterol moving from the liver to the cells or arteries.

What we'll be talking about in this section is crucial because, even though you might be worried if your LDL is extremely high, when you see the doctor to get your cholesterol checked, they almost always only test your LDL cholesterol and don't examine anything else that might be related to it. Since a very specific sort of LDL and a test that you would have to request are the true villains in the story of cholesterol and heart problems, it is crucial to realize that there are two different measurements for LDL.

This test, which stands for LDLP particle which is an Advanced Lipid Profile Test, will display the quantity and size of the particles. What is a particle, then? There are two particle sizes of LDL, the large buoyant version is called "pattern A," and buoyant means it floats to the surface. As was previously stated, it is a carrier that moves this cholesterol because it needs to have this protein little capsule to transport it. Therefore, it is these large fluffy particles that are floating through the bloodstream carrying cholesterol.

Then there are the little, dense particles that can get inside an artery since the inside of an artery is only around the thickness of a single cell. This is where the difficulty lies. The pathogenic LDL, not the huge buoyant LDL, but the small dense LDL, is where the issue originates. The key reason for concern should be the small dense LDL. The question I want to ask you at this point is, which LDL do you think has higher cholesterol? If you guessed large buoyant, you are right, so if your blood work results show that your LDL cholesterol is high, that information doesn't reveal what kind of particles you have more of.

It primarily provides information on the total amount of cholesterol, though some people with low levels of LDL cholesterol also have higher concentrations of the small, dense LVL particles, and many others with high levels of LDL cholesterol also have higher concentrations of the large, buoyant pattern type of LDL. Because it will offer you a complete view of what is happening, insist on receiving this Advanced Lipid Profile Test whenever you have your cholesterol examined.

Which Cholesterol-Rich Foods Should I Avoid?

Fast food

Regular consumption of fast food increases the chance of developing chronic diseases like obesity, diabetes, and heart disease.

Fast food also raises the risk of excessive levels of inflammation, abdominal fat, heart disease, and blood sugar regulation.

Processed meats

You should stay clear of processed meats like bacon, sausages, and hot dogs in your diet.

If processed meat consumption is not restricted, it can lead to colon cancer and heart problems.

Fried food

Fried meals are mostly linked to low-density lipoprotein (LDL), or poor cholesterol.

Trans fat

Trans fats and its high calorie content contribute to heart disease, diabetes, and obesity.

Vegetable oil solidifies at room temperature when hydrogen is added, which results in the formation of trans fats.

Food prepared with hydrogenated oil has a longer shelf life because this procedure is typically carried out by businesses, which makes hydrogenated oil less expensive and less prone to spoil.

Because it won't need to be changed as frequently as other oils, the majority of restaurants utilize it in their deep fryers.

Small levels of trans fat are present in several dairy and meat products.

Trans fat can be found in a variety of food products:

- Commercially baked foods (cakes, pies, and cookies).
- Shortening
- Microwave popcorn
- Frozen pizza
- Refrigerated dough (biscuits and rolls)

- Fried foods (French fries, doughnuts, and fried chicken)
- Nondairy coffee creamer
- Stick margarine etc...

Small dense lipoprotein (LDL)

Now let's briefly go over more information regarding this tiny dense LDL, which is shown on your blood profile as "sdLDL." The first thing you should be aware of is that you will have higher levels of this profile—small dense LDL (sdLDL)—if you have metabolic syndrome, insulin resistance, obesity, or diabetes. You may also see this pattern—as was previously mentioned—if you have lower levels of LDLC cholesterol. Here, we are not evaluating the particles themselves but rather the cholesterol **inside** of these particles. This is crucial information for you to be aware of because there is sdLDL.

The tiny dense form of LDL that is involved in glycation is the atherogenic LDL. The term "glycation" basically refers to the process of mixing a protein with sugar, which renders the protein non-functional and causes issues with the proteins lining your arteries. Additionally, this type of measurement is connected to oxidation, which is another factor associated with inflammation and free radical damage. a favorable environment for the spread of bacteria, the formation of biofilms, tissue removal, and a cascade of other events, however, in addition to plaque buildup in your arteries, you frequently have biofilms, which are essentially microorganisms in calcium shells that tend to collect on the rough edges of your arteries brought on by oxidation or inflammation. As a result, small dense LDL is a strong 3x predictor of cardiovascular disease.

The other intriguing aspect of this is that while statin medications will lower your cholesterol, they do not affect this small dense LDL; in fact, they may even increase it. The main issue at hand is how to precisely lower the genuine bad LDL, which is the small dense version.

The best food to lower cholesterol

Well, there are some things you may consume that will benefit you. Each of the meals that will be mentioned has a considerable reducing effect on the tiny dense LDL, and they are all completely researched and proven foods.

Dr. Eric Berg DC, an internist with more than 20 years of experience in Solomons, Maryland, and an affiliate with Calvert Health Medical Center, as well as the author of the best-selling book The Healthy Keto Plan and the Director of Dr. Berg Nutritionals, recommends the following foods in a YouTube video:

two avocados, because they are high in healthy fat, an extra virgin olive oil that you must make sure, is the real thing because there are many fake extra virgin olive oils out there. The following oil is fish oil, particularly cod liver oil, though you can also utilize fish oils. The omega-3 fatty acids, which include both EPA and DHA, come next; it appears that EPA is the one that has this reducing effect.

The next food is pistachios, which have also been shown to lower this small dense LDL. Next is dark chocolate, of which I would always recommend the sugar-free variety.

Finally, there are almonds, which have also been shown to lower this tiny dense lipoprotein. Lastly, walnuts can aid in lowering harmful cholesterol.

Other natural ways to lower cholesterol

There are a few other pretty fascinating things that have to do with this subject as well. One of them is "Niacin," in particular the kind of niacin that induces blushing and has the power to transform from one particle size to another. These indicate that it can change your LDL cholesterol slightly lower while also switching from the small dense LDL to the large buoyant LDL, which is very good.

The next thing you could do is exercise, which will undoubtedly also help to lower this small dense LDL. If your problem is particularly stubborn, you could also try "Tudca," a very specific bile salt that helps the body get rid of extra cholesterol, Include extra exercise in your everyday routine by using the stairs instead of the elevator, parking farther from your workplace, going for a walk during breaks or downtime, and standing up more while doing chores like cooking or yard work.

You should also be aware that bile salts regulate cholesterol in the body bile salts are made from cholesterol, so if you are lacking in bile, such as if you have a fatty liver or no gallbladder, or if you have eaten foods that have slowed down the function of your bile ducts, that may be the cause of your high cholesterol. In this case, you should start taking bile salts, especially if you have a genetic condition that causes high cholesterol.

Please note, if you do have a genetic problem with your cholesterol and you want to do the ketogenic diet which I highly recommend with fasting, the thing you would want to do is not necessarily completely go low fat, you just want to avoid the extra fat that a lot of people take on the ketogenic diet which means you would not want to take the extra MCT oil and also don't want to start consuming the keto bomb treats filled with fat and butter, but you do want to increase the fish oils and the fish because that is not going to increase your problem. Additionally, sugar, especially fructose, is the worst food to consume because it tends to make problems worse.

This goes for all refined carbohydrates as well. Look for a means to quit smoking, these have immediate health benefits since it raises HDL (good) cholesterol levels. Your blood pressure and heart rate return to normal shortly after quitting cigarettes. Additionally, you will note that as your blood circulates, and your lung function improves over time, your risk of developing heart disease will vanish.

Although it is claimed that moderate alcohol consumption is associated with higher levels of HDL (good) cholesterol, this association does not support the recommendation of alcohol for non-drinkers.

Serious health issues like high blood pressure, heart failure, or a stroke can result from excessive alcohol consumption. Small weight loss adjustments add up to big results because being overweight raises cholesterol levels. If you typically consume sugary beverages, try switching to water.

If you are curious to know how fasting can be your main strategy against cancerous cells, then search for "fasting; your main strategy against cancer, by Julius Abdul" on Amazon, and discover how fasting and another diet strategy can help prevent or cure cancer.

Conclusion

LDL is considered bad cholesterol, while HDL is considered good. However, there are two kinds of LDL. A specific type of LDL is the true villain when it comes to cholesterol and heart disease.

To measure this type of LDL, you must request a test known as an advanced lipid profile test. They are looking at the number and size of the particles that carry cholesterol with this test.

LDL is classified into two types or particle sizes which are; the massive buoyant (pattern A) and the tiny dense (pattern B).

Even though the large buoyant type carries more cholesterol, the small dense LDL particles are the ones to be concerned about because they can enter the arteries. Small dense LDL cholesterol is an excellent predictor of cardiovascular disease, because some people have low LDL cholesterol but a high number of small dense particles, this topic can be perplexing.

Others have high LDL and a lot of large buoyant particles. This is why it's critical to get an advanced lipid profile test to get a complete picture of what's going on.

Extra virgin olive oil, avocados, fish oils or cod liver oil, pistachios, dark chocolate (sugar-free), almonds, and walnuts are the top foods that lower bad cholesterol (small dense LDL).

Other natural ways to lower cholesterol include taking vitamin B3 (niacin), exercising, and taking TUDCA.

Simple Ideas For A Healthy Lifestyle

Eat good food, and by that I mean a balanced diet, a little bit of everything is not bad, but too much of everything is the opposite.

Always drink water even when you don't want to. Staying hydrated is a big boost to body metabolism (digestion and conversion of food to energy).

Keeping fit through regular exercise will not only burn your body fat and keep you in good shape but will also give you the ability to control your body. Remember how good it feels when you are in control.

Stress is the number one boost to different ailments in the body and if you have a phobia of falling sick, which I believe every reasonable human being do, then you must manage stress by having a **good sleep and rest**.

If I have super powers I will stop you from taking alcohol, but since I'm a human being like you and I know how we can be addicted to some lifestyle characteristics, then I'll advise you to **reduce your alcohol intake** because it doesn't only affect your system, but also lead to accident and injuries.

Stop smoking, smoking is more dangerous than number 5 above because it targets the heart, and whatever stops the heart from functioning, you know the rest of the story. Smokers are liable to die young, these brands do not hide it from you! What else do you want?

Do not expose yourself to any external and environmental threats to health like hazards, toxins, and rays like the sun.

Cutting your nails and washing your hands is an easy practice but saves you a lot. Long nails are a haven for bacteria that can be transferred to anything your hands come in contact with, also if you are in the 2020s, coronavirus! Please, wash your hands.

Can you remember this monster called sex urge? It is one of the fastest transmitters of diseases, for your health's sake, **practice safe sex by using condoms.**

PS: I am confident that you have acquired a lot of
value from this Book.

I adore you and wish you luck on your new journey.

I'll see you at the top of your health.